FROM MANAGING TO CONQUERING GENITAL GENITAL HERPES

Expert Guide To Understanding the Causes, Recognizing Symptoms, Prevention and Embracing Effective Treatments for a Vibrant and Healthy Life

DR. DASHIELL DANIEL

THE VIROLOGY OF HERPES VULGARIS 12
DYNAMICS OF TRANSMISSION 13
CLINICAL DISPLAY 13
IDENTIFICATION AND LABORATORY EVALUATION 14
CONTROL AND INTERVENTION 15
STRATEGIES FOR PREVENTION 16
PSYCHOSOCIAL REPERCUSSIONS 17
CONSIDERING PUBLIC HEALTH 17
CHAPTER ONE COMPREHENDING GENITAL HERPES 20

CHAPTER TWO 24

INDICATIONS AND SYMPTOMS 24

CHAPTER THREE 30

DIAGNOSIS AND TESTING 30
CLINICAL ASSESSMENT 30
TESTS IN THE LAB 31
POLYMERASE CHAIN REACTION (PCR) 32
TESTS FOR BLOOD 32
DIAGNOSIS'S PSYCHOLOGICAL EFFECTS 33

CHAPTER FOUR 35

POSSIBLE TREATMENTS 35

CHAPTER FIVE 39

PREVENTION STRATEGIES 39
SAFE PROCEDURES 39
ABSTINENCE 39

RESEARCH AND VACCINES   40
CURRENT DEVELOPMENTS IN VACCINES   41
CLINICAL EXAMINATIONS   42

CHAPTER SIX   **44**

LIVING WITH GENITAL HERPES   **44**
ASPECTS OF EMOTION AND PSYCHOLOGY   44
ADAPTIVE TECHNIQUES   45
ASSISTANCE NETWORKS   45
RELATIONSHIPS AND DISCLOSURE   46
SPEAKING WITH PARTNERS   46
INTIMACY AND DATING   47
FAQS REGARDING GENITAL HERPES   48
CAN YOU CURE GENITAL HERPES?   49
WHAT IMPACT DOES GENITAL HERPES HAVE ON CONCEPTION?   50
DO SEXUALLY TRANSMITTED DISEASES (STDS) INCLUDE HERPES?   51

CHAPTER EIGHT   **53**

FALLACIES AND MISUNDERSTANDINGS   **53**
ORAL SEX AND HERPES   53
RESTROOM SEATS AND HERPES   54
HERPES AND INFORMAL INTERACTION   55

CHAPTER NINE   **58**

PROSPECTIVE ROUTES   **58**
IMPROVEMENTS IN MEDICAL CARE   59
ADVANCES IN VACCINATION   61
AWARENESS AND ADVOCACY   63
CONCLUSION   **64**

Disclaimer

This book, is intended to provide information and guidance on the subject matter and is not a substitute for professional medical advice, diagnosis, or treatment.

The author, is not a medical professional, and the content presented here is based on research, general knowledge, and expert guidance available at the time of writing.

The information in this book is provided with the understanding that the author and the publisher are not engaged in rendering medical, legal, or other professional services.

Any reliance on the information contained in this book is at the reader's own risk.

While every effort has been made to ensure the accuracy and completeness of the information presented, medical knowledge is constantly evolving, and new research may supersede the content in this book. The author and the publisher make no representations or warranties of any kind, express or implied, about the completeness, accuracy, reliability, suitability, or availability concerning the information, products, services, or related graphics contained in this book.

This book may contain references or mentions of individuals, products, websites, organizations, or other names for informational purposes only.

The author does not own or endorse any such entities mentioned in the book. Any resemblance to actual persons, living or dead, or actual events is purely coincidental.

Readers are encouraged to consult with qualified healthcare professionals for medical advice, diagnosis, and treatment tailored to their specific circumstances.

The author and the publisher disclaim any liability for any loss or risk, personal or otherwise, arising directly or indirectly from the use of the information presented in this book.

By reading this book, the reader acknowledges and agrees to the terms of this disclaimer.

The book "Genital Herpes" is an all-inclusive manual for comprehending, handling, and negotiating the intricacies associated with this common sexually transmitted infection (STI).

The book begins by outlining the general significance of bringing genital herpes to light, stressing how common it is and how important it is to fully comprehend all of its facets. The content is organized in a way that provides readers with the necessary knowledge, highlighting the importance of awareness, prevention, and support for those who are impacted by genital herpes.

The first chapter gives a basic overview of genital herpes, including its definition, the different kinds of herpes viruses, and the main causes and ways in which it is spread. The following chapters examine various aspects of the infection in detail, including symptoms, diagnosis techniques, available treatments, and preventative measures. This methodical approach guarantees that the reader obtains a sophisticated understanding of the complex nature of genital herpes.

The book's thorough examination of the psychological and emotional effects of a genital herpes diagnosis, with a focus on coping mechanisms and the value of support systems, is one of its most notable features.

The book discusses the infection's wider effects on dating, intimacy, and relationships in addition to its clinical components.

In-depth chapters that disprove myths and answer commonly asked questions (FAQs) about genital herpes help to eliminate misinformation and promote more informed public discourse.

The book also discusses ongoing research, therapeutic developments, vaccination breakthroughs, and the necessity of ongoing activism and awareness as it looks to the future.

"Genital Herpes" offers a comprehensive and perceptive examination of the condition that goes beyond the traditional medical discourse.

It is an invaluable tool for researchers, healthcare professionals, people with genital herpes, and the general public. It advances our understanding of this common STI and opens the door to better advocacy, management, and prevention. Introduction:

The herpes simplex virus (HSV) is the common sexually transmitted infection (STI) that causes genital herpes. The development of painful sores or blisters around the vaginal and anal regions is the defining feature of this illness.

HSV-1 and HSV-2 are the two primary HSV kinds that cause genital herpes; the former is typically linked to oral herpes, while the latter is primarily associated with genital infections. Millions of people worldwide are impacted by genital herpes, which poses difficulties for diagnosis, treatment, and prevention.

1. An overview of herpes genital:

A persistent, recurrent infection, genital herpes has a substantial negative influence on the physical and mental health of those who have it.

The virus causes sporadic symptom outbursts by establishing latency in nerve cells. Asymptomatic shedding can happen in between episodes, which helps spread the virus. During outbreaks, the clinical presentation may include painful sores, itching, and flu-like symptoms. Genital herpes has a complicated epidemiology, with varied prevalence rates in various demographic groups and geographical areas. Effective prevention, diagnosis, and treatment of genital herpes require a thorough understanding of the virology, dynamics of transmission, and clinical characteristics of the condition.

2. Objective of the Book:

This book aims to give readers a thorough and reliable resource on genital herpes by addressing many facets of the virus from a multidisciplinary standpoint.

It seeks to close the knowledge gap between research findings, clinical expertise, and general public understanding. Through the integration of data from clinical medicine, epidemiology, virology, and public health, the book aims to provide insightful analysis for medical professionals, researchers, teachers, and the general public. Enhancing knowledge of genital herpes, busting myths, and advancing evidence-based methods for diagnosis, treatment, and prevention are the objectives.

3. Understanding Genital Herpes Is Crucial

Because of its extensive prevalence, influence on reproductive health, and associated problems, understanding genital herpes is essential.

The illness affects psychological and emotional health as well as sexual and reproductive decisions. Furthermore, the significance of genital herpes for public health is highlighted by its role in promoting the spread of other STIs, such as HIV. Healthcare professionals must possess a thorough grasp of genital herpes in order to give correct information, appropriate counseling, and successful preventative efforts. Furthermore, in order to lower stigma, support testing, and encourage safe sexual behavior—all of which improve community health—public knowledge is essential.

The Virology Of Herpes Vulgaris

Two closely related viruses, HSV-1 and HSV-2, both members of the Herpesviridae family, are the main cause of genital herpes. These viruses have a special capacity to infect sensory nerve ganglia and create latent infections, which can periodically reactivate and cause repeated clinical symptoms. The pathophysiology of genital herpes is largely determined by the structure, replication cycle, and interactions of the virus with host cells. Comprehending the virology of genital herpes is essential for creating vaccines, therapeutic interventions, and antiviral tactics.

Dynamics Of Transmission

Genital herpes is distributed through a variety of intricate and varied mechanisms. The most typical method of transmission is through sexual contact with infected vaginal, oral, or anal mucosa. It is also possible for there to be vertical transfer from mother to child during birthing, which might have very serious effects on the newborn. Furthermore, viral transmission is aided by shedding of the virus when no symptoms are present. To stop the spread of genital herpes, it is essential to understand these transmission dynamics in order to put preventive measures into place, counsel afflicted individuals, and create public health campaigns.

Clinical Display

Genital herpes can present clinically in a variety of ways, from an asymptomatic infection to severe, recurring outbreaks.

The traditional presentation consists of excruciating genital blisters or ulcers, along with systemic symptoms as fever and malaise. Diagnosis is difficult, nevertheless, because unusual presentations and subclinical illnesses are frequent. In order to correctly diagnose and treat genital herpes, healthcare professionals must have a thorough understanding of the many clinical symptoms. It also highlights the necessity of a patient-centered, multifaceted approach to care that takes into account each person's particular experiences and difficulties related to the infection.

Identification And Laboratory Evaluation

A combination of scientific testing and clinical evaluation is needed to diagnose genital herpes. Viral culture, polymerase chain reaction (PCR), and serological assays are among the diagnostic techniques that are essential for verifying the existence of HSV and differentiating between HSV-1 and HSV-2 infections.

Accurate diagnosis requires understanding the limitations of each testing method, interpreting test results, and taking sample collection timing into account. Healthcare professionals may customize treatment strategies and give appropriate counseling to patients diagnosed with genital herpes thanks to the integration of clinical and laboratory data.

Control And Intervention

A multimodal strategy involving antiviral drugs, supportive care, and counseling is used to manage genital herpes. The majority of treatment is antiviral medication, such as acyclovir, valacyclovir, and famciclovir, which aims to relieve symptoms, inhibit viral shedding, and lessen the severity and duration of outbreaks.

Antiviral medication works well, but it does not eliminate the virus, which emphasizes the need for continued medical care and psychological support. Comprehensive care must include counseling on safe sexual behavior, disclosing to partners, and managing the emotional effects of genital herpes.

Strategies For Prevention

A mix of behavioral treatments, education, and maybe vaccination is used to prevent genital herpes. Promoting safer sexual behaviors lowers the risk of sexual transmission, such as consistent and appropriate condom usage.

Prevention initiatives benefit from education campaigns that highlight the significance of routine testing, early diagnosis, and treatment.

Research on the creation of a herpes vaccine is ongoing and could offer long-term defense against HSV infection.

In order to lessen the prevalence of genital herpes and its effects on people and communities, it is essential to comprehend and put these preventive techniques into practice.

Psychosocial Repercussions

Beyond its physical manifestations, genital herpes has a psychosocial impact that impacts relationships, mental health, and general quality of life. Misconceptions and stigma related to the virus might cause emotions of guilt, loneliness, and fear. For those with genital herpes, communicating the diagnosis to sexual partners and negotiating the complexities of intimate relationships present serious obstacles. In order to address the psychosocial elements of the infection, provide support, and make counseling services more accessible, healthcare providers are essential.

A comprehensive approach to patient care must acknowledge and treat the psychological effects of genital herpes.

Considering Public Health

Because genital herpes has a significant impact on public health, preventative and control strategies must be integrated and grounded in research.

The main goals of public health initiatives should be to increase knowledge, lessen stigma, and support sexual health education. Genital herpes can be prevented and detected early with the use of routine testing, targeted therapies for high-risk populations, and accessible, reasonably priced healthcare. Furthermore, integrated public health activities are crucial given the role that genital herpes plays in enabling the transmission of other STIs, including HIV. Public health programs must be developed and implemented in concert with legislators, healthcare professionals, and community stakeholders.

To sum up, genital herpes is a serious public health issue that affects both people and communities widely. The numerous aspects of genital herpes are thoroughly explored in this book, including its virology, dynamics of transmission, clinical presentation, diagnosis, treatment, prevention, psychosocial effects, and public health implications.

Multidisciplinary knowledge on genital herpes is crucial for medical professionals, researchers, teachers, and the general public.

This book supports coordinated efforts to lessen the burden of genital herpes and enhance general sexual and reproductive health by providing factual information, busting myths, and advocating evidence-based practices.

CHAPTER ONE
COMPREHENDING GENITAL HERPES

The herpes simplex virus (HSV) is the common sexually transmitted infection (STI) that causes genital herpes. This virus mainly affects the anal and vaginal regions, resulting in blisters and painful sores. HSV-1 and HSV-2 are the two primary herpes viral types that cause genital herpes. HSV-1 can lead to genital herpes through oral-genital contact, even though it is the typical source of oral herpes. On the other hand, the majority of genital herpes cases are mostly caused by HSV-2. The infection is a chronic illness that has no known cure, and it is typified by painful sore eruptions that occur repeatedly.

A member of the Herpesviridae family, the herpes simplex virus (HSV) is well-known for its capacity to cause latent infections in the nerve cells of its host. Given that HSV-1 and HSV-2 are highly contagious and can spread through a variety of channels, it is essential to comprehend how they spread and what causes them in order to develop effective preventative measures.

The double-stranded DNA virus known as Herpes Simplex Virus (HSV) comes in two different serotypes: HSV-1 and HSV-2. These viruses develop latency in sensory nerve ganglia and mainly infect mucosal surfaces, including the vaginal and oral areas. HSV-2 is the main virus that causes genital herpes, whereas HSV-1 is frequently linked to oral lesions. Although the viruses' preferred anatomical locations and modes of transmission differ, they have structural similarities.

A major factor in the spread of genital herpes is the modes of transmission. The main method of transmission is direct contact with contaminated vaginal, oral, or anal secretions. Both vaginal and anal sex provide a significant risk of virus transmission, particularly when there are current outbreaks and greater virus concentrations.

Other possible routes of HSV infection include sharing of personal belongings, oral-genital contact, and vertical transfer from mother to child during birthing. It is essential to comprehend these modes in order to put preventive measures into action.

Risk factors for genital herpes can take many different forms, such as immune system function, sexual behavior, and demographics.

The chance of contracting genital herpes is greatly increased when engaging in unprotected sexual activity with an infected partner. The risk is further increased by multiple sexual partners, compromised immune systems, and high-risk activities. Age and gender are two further demographic characteristics that come into play, with women and young individuals being more vulnerable. Moreover, those who have previously had other STDs may be more susceptible to developing genital herpes.

Education, alterations in behavior, and occasionally antiviral drugs are used to stop the spread of genital herpes. The risk of transmission can be greatly decreased by using condoms correctly and consistently as part of safe sexual practices. The management and prevention of genital herpes necessitate early symptom diagnosis, timely medical action, and communication between sexual partners. Though there is presently no publicly accessible vaccine for genital herpes, vaccination research is ongoing.

a thorough comprehension of genital herpes necessitates investigating the definition and fundamentals of the illness, investigating the complexities of the herpes simplex virus, scrutinizing the diverse means of transmission, and pinpointing the correlated risk factors.

This information is essential for creating preventative plans that work, encouraging safer sexual behaviors, and eventually lowering the incidence and consequences of genital herpes in people all over the world.

CHAPTER TWO
INDICATIONS AND SYMPTOMS

The herpes simplex virus (HSV) is the source of genital herpes, a sexually transmitted infection (STI). There are two forms of the virus: HSV-1, which is usually linked to oral herpes, and HSV-2, which is frequently tied to genital herpes.

The signs and symptoms of genital herpes will be thoroughly covered in this discussion, including the condition's duration and severity, main symptoms, lesions and sores, pain and discomfort, recurrent symptoms, and triggers for outbreaks.

Primary genital herpes symptoms appear during the first infection and are frequently more noticeable than recurring symptoms. Lesions or sores on the genitalia and adjacent areas arise during the main outbreak. Along with other flu-like symptoms including fever, headache, and swollen lymph nodes, these sores can be painful and irritating. Individuals may experience varying degrees of discomfort from the primary symptoms; some may just experience minor discomfort, while others may experience more severe manifestations. Comprehending the unique characteristics of initial symptoms is essential for prompt diagnosis and suitable therapy.

Genital herpes is characterized by lesions and sores, which can occur in both initial and recurrent outbreaks. Usually tiny, fluid-filled blisters, the sores have the potential to ulcerate and become uncomfortable open sores. These sores are extremely contagious and can transfer the virus to other people when they come into direct touch with one another. Furthermore, the development of lesions may worsen the psychological effects of genital herpes, depressing the afflicted person and lowering their quality of life. The goal of management techniques is frequently to reduce the discomfort brought on by these obvious signs.

Genital herpes is characterized by pain and discomfort, which can impact both initial and recurring outbreaks. Genital herpes can cause moderate to severe pain, which can negatively affect everyday activities and quality of life. Activities like urination, sexual relations, and other physical movements might make discomfort worse. An important part of treating genital herpes is addressing pain and discomfort, which frequently entails using antiviral drugs, analgesics, and topical therapies to lessen symptoms and improve the quality of life for those who are impacted.

After the first outbreak, genital herpes symptoms are frequently recurrent. Lesions and sores tend to return during future outbreaks, despite the original episode typically being more severe. Individual differences exist in the frequency and severity of recurring outbreaks; some may have mild, rare recurrences, while others may have more frequent, severe episodes. The physical and emotional elements of genital herpes require continuous management and assistance due to recurrent symptoms, which can exacerbate the condition's long-term difficulties.

The recurrence of genital herpes symptoms is significantly influenced by triggers for outbreaks. Lesions and sores may appear as a result of the virus being activated by a number of different conditions. Stress, disease, hormone fluctuations, and specific lifestyle elements are common triggers. For those who are treating genital herpes, knowing what causes them is crucial because lifestyle changes and stress-reduction tactics can reduce the frequency and intensity of outbreaks.

In addition, medical professionals can provide direction on identifying and addressing any triggers, which can improve the condition's overall management.

The length and intensity of herpes infections in the genitalia might differ greatly between people. Recurrent outbreaks typically occur for shorter periods of time than the first episode, which typically lasts longer and is more intense. Numerous variables, including the patient's general health, the functioning of their immune system, and the timely administration of medication, might impact the intensity of symptoms during a recurrence. While some people may only see a few breakouts throughout their lifetime, others might deal with more frequent recurrences. In the long-term management of genital herpes, controlling the length and intensity of outbreaks is crucial, highlighting the significance of individualized treatment regimens and continuing medical supervision.

Conclusively, a thorough comprehension of the indications and manifestations of genital herpes is imperative for efficient handling and assistance. Lesions, sores, soreness, and discomfort are examples of primary symptoms that shed light on the early stages of an infection, whereas repeated symptoms emphasize the chronic character of the illness. A comprehensive strategy to treating genital herpes involves determining the factors that lead to outbreaks as well as managing the length and intensity of symptoms. Through the integration of medical interventions, lifestyle modifications, and psychological support, healthcare practitioners can enable persons impacted by genital herpes to effectively manage the obstacles linked to this common and significant sexually transmitted infection.

CHAPTER THREE
DIAGNOSIS AND TESTING

Genital herpes diagnosis and testing entails a thorough process that includes laboratory testing, clinical evaluation, and recognition of the psychological effects of the diagnosis.

Clinical Assessment

A crucial part of diagnosing genital herpes is a clinical examination. Getting a thorough medical history from patients is usually the first step taken by healthcare providers. This includes learning about the patient's sexual history and any prior genital lesion incidents. During the physical examination, the genital region is closely inspected for sores, ulcers, or any other obvious indications. The inspection could also cover nearby regions like the thighs and buttocks. Additionally, doctors evaluate the patient for indications of a systemic ailment. An accurate preliminary diagnosis is made easier by this comprehensive approach, which helps identify distinctive clinical symptoms such vesicles, ulcers, and regional lymphadenopathy.

Tests In The Lab

Particularly in cases when clinical presentations are ambiguous or unusual, laboratory investigations are essential for verifying the diagnosis of genital herpes. A highly sensitive and specific diagnostic technique for identifying viral DNA in clinical specimens is polymerase chain reaction (PCR) (3.2.1). Herpes simplex virus (HSV) DNA is amplified and identified using this molecular method, which yields a conclusive diagnosis. By looking for antibodies against HSV, blood tests (3.2.2) such serological assays assist in assessing the patient's immunological response. Blood tests are useful for determining the stage of infection (primary versus recurrent) and for differentiating between HSV-1 and HSV-2 infections, even though PCR is crucial for early infection identification. When combined, these lab tests support a thorough diagnosis process.

Polymerase Chain Reaction (Pcr)

The molecular biology method known as PCR has completely changed how genital herpes is diagnosed. Viral DNA is amplified and detected using this extremely sensitive and specific approach, which offers a quick and precise diagnosis. PCR testing is performed on clinical specimens, such as swabs from genital lesions or cerebral fluid in cases of suspected meningitis. The test determines the particular type of herpes simplex virus (HSV-1 or HSV-2) in addition to confirming its existence. Early on in an infection, when viral shedding is high but clinical signs may be mild, PCR is especially helpful. Because of its accuracy, it is a vital tool for prompt intervention and suitable patient care.

Tests For Blood

Blood tests are essential to the diagnosis of genital herpes because they help distinguish between HSV-1 and HSV-2 infections and provide information on the patient's immune response. Antibodies against HSV are found in the patient's blood by serological techniques such the Western blot and enzyme-linked immunosorbent assay (ELISA). IgG antibodies show immunity from prior exposure, whereas IgM antibodies indicate a recent infection. Clinicians are able to detect infections and ascertain the stage and probability of recurrence by combining PCR and blood tests. These tests help determine the best course of treatment and provide a thorough picture of the patient's infection status.

Diagnosis's Psychological Effects

Genital herpes diagnoses have a profound psychological impact on patients, in addition to their medical symptoms. A person may experience a variety of feelings after learning about a sexually transmitted virus, such as shame, remorse, worry, and anxiety. Healthcare professionals must comprehend the psychological effects in order to give comprehensive care. The stigma attached to genital herpes can have a negative impact on mental health and frequently cause feelings of isolation. Support groups and counseling are essential in assisting patients in overcoming the psychological difficulties brought on by their illness. Psychological components must be addressed in order to support general well-being, make treatment plans easier to follow, and avoid problems that could arise from stress and mental health.

genital herpes testing and diagnosis require a multimodal strategy that combines laboratory testing like PCR and blood tests with clinical evaluation. This all-encompassing approach facilitates prompt and precise infection diagnosis, supporting suitable patient care. Furthermore, it is critical to acknowledge the psychological ramifications of a genital herpes diagnosis in order to provide comprehensive care and attend to the emotional health of those afflicted with this STD.

CHAPTER FOUR
POSSIBLE TREATMENTS

The herpes simplex virus is the source of genital herpes, a sexually transmitted infection (HSV). While there isn't a cure for this chronic illness, there are a number of treatment methods that try to control symptoms and lessen the frequency and intensity of outbreaks. We will examine the main genital herpes treatment options in this talk, with an emphasis on antiviral drugs, controlling outbreaks, over-the-counter medicines, and lifestyle modifications.

The mainstay of treatment for genital herpes is antiviral drugs, which work by inhibiting the herpes simplex virus to reduce symptoms. One common antiviral drug prescribed for genital herpes is acyclovir. It lessens the intensity and duration of outbreaks by blocking the process of viral DNA replication. The availability of acyclovir in oral, topical, and injectable formulations offers a range of therapy alternatives.

An additional antiviral drug used to treat genital herpes is valacyclovir. It is a prodrug of acyclovir, which means that the body changes it into acyclovir. Because valacyclovir has a longer half-life than acyclovir, it provides the benefit of requiring fewer doses. This makes it an easy option for anyone looking for a more convenient way to take their medications while still successfully suppressing the herpes virus.

A third effective antiviral treatment for genital herpes is famciclovir. The body also changes it into penciclovir, which is its active form.

When treating recurrent genital herpes outbreaks, famciclovir is especially helpful. It can be given as a single-day, high-dose treatment to hasten healing.

The availability of several antiviral drugs gives medical practitioners the flexibility to customize treatment regimens to meet the specific needs and preferences of each patient.

Another important part of treating genital herpes is controlling outbreaks. In addition to antiviral drugs, home remedies can provide symptom alleviation and enhance general health. Pain and inflammation related to genital herpes lesions can be reduced by localized applications of ice or cold compresses. Additionally, in order to stop subsequent bacterial infections and encourage quicker healing, it's critical to keep up good hygiene practices in the affected area.

Modifying one's lifestyle is essential for controlling genital herpes and lowering breakout frequency. Since stress can either cause or worsen outbreaks, stress management is essential. Including stress-relieving practices in one's lifestyle, such as yoga, meditation, and regular exercise, can help the condition progress more favorably. Getting enough sleep is also essential because sleep deprivation impairs immunity and increases the risk of herpes breakouts.

In addition, it's critical for people with genital herpes to change to safer sexual behaviors in order to stop the virus from spreading to potential partners. Although condom use is not 100%

protective, it can dramatically lower the risk of transmission when done correctly and consistently. It is essential to be open and honest with sexual partners about the illness in order to promote awareness and a sense of shared responsibility for stopping its spread.

genital herpes therapy entails a multimodal strategy that combines antiviral drugs, controlling outbreaks using homemade therapies, and altering lifestyle choices. Personalized treatment plans are made possible by the availability of a variety of antiviral drugs, and avoidance of outbreaks and general well-being are enhanced by home remedies and lifestyle modifications. When these methods are combined, it offers genital herpes patients a holistic plan that supports their mental and physical well-being.

CHAPTER FIVE
PREVENTION STRATEGIES
Safe Procedures

The prevention of genital herpes, a sexually transmitted infection brought on by the herpes simplex virus (HSV), is mostly dependent on safe practices. One key safe practice that has received a lot of support is the usage of condoms. By acting as a barrier, condoms lower the possibility of HSV transmission during sex. It's crucial to remember that condoms might not offer total protection because HSV might infect places that they don't cover. However, using condoms correctly and consistently is still a crucial part of safe practices for preventing genital herpes.

Abstinence

One of the most important preventative measures against genital herpes is abstinence, or choosing not to engage in sexual activity. Since sexual contact is the primary means of transmission of HSV, refraining from sexual activity reduces the chance of infection. Those who are not in monogamous partnerships or who are uncertain of their partner's HSV status are especially encouraged to abstain. Abstinence is still a safe option for people who want to completely eliminate the chance of genital herpes transmission, even though it may not be a desirable or realistic decision for everyone.

Research And Vaccines

Research into vaccine development to prevent genital herpes has been ongoing. Vaccines work to prevent or lessen the severity of infection by boosting the immune system's ability to identify and fight the herpes simplex virus. Several strategies are being used in the current vaccine development process, such as live attenuated vaccines and subunit vaccinations. By focusing on particular viral components, these vaccines stimulate the immune system without actually spreading the illness. It is crucial to comprehend both the host reaction and the immunology of HSV while developing vaccinations.

Current Developments In Vaccines

There are currently a number of vaccine candidates for genital herpes prevention in varying stages of development. These candidates usually concentrate on glycoproteins like gD and gB that are present on the surface of the herpes simplex virus. These glycoproteins are essential for the virus's ability to enter host cells. Researchers hope to develop vaccines that can drive the development of neutralizing antibodies, so blocking the entry of viruses and preventing illness, by focusing on these components.

There is hope that a genital herpes vaccine that is both widely available and effective will eventually be developed because to advancements in vaccine development.

Clinical Examinations

When assessing the safety and effectiveness of prospective genital herpes vaccines, clinical trials are essential. The purpose of these meticulously planned trials, which involve human subjects, is to evaluate the vaccine's effectiveness in regulated settings. The stages of clinical trials offer a standardized framework for vaccine development, ranging from large-scale efficacy trials to early-phase safety research. Clinical trial participants' side effects, immunological responses, and overall vaccine efficacy are tracked. A genital herpes vaccine's successful completion of clinical trials is a necessary step toward regulatory approval and ultimately general distribution.

genital herpes prevention entails a multimodal strategy that includes safe practices, abstinence, and continued vaccination research.

The encouraging advancements in vaccine research provide promise for a more comprehensive and long-term solution to lower the prevalence of genital herpes, while safe practices like condom usage and abstinence serve as immediate preventive measures. Clinical trials are essential to converting scientific discoveries into practical preventive measures and laying the groundwork for a time when highly efficient vaccines will greatly reduce the spread of genital herpes.

CHAPTER SIX
LIVING WITH GENITAL HERPES

The herpes simplex virus (HSV) is the source of genital herpes, a sexually transmitted infection (STI). People with genital herpes frequently deal with a variety of emotional and physical difficulties. This section delves into the psychological and emotional elements of having genital herpes, discussing coping mechanisms and the value of social support systems.

Aspects Of Emotion And Psychology

A diagnosis of genital herpes can have a significant emotional and psychological impact. A variety of emotions, such as astonishment, fear, wrath, and grief, may be felt by individuals. Dealing with the stigma attached to herpes can be especially difficult. Coping mechanisms are essential for assisting people in overcoming the psychological effects of having genital herpes.

Adaptive Techniques

Having good coping mechanisms in place is crucial to controlling the psychological effects of genital herpes. Reframing unfavorable ideas and engaging in mindfulness exercises are two cognitive-behavioral techniques that can support the development of resilience in people. Seeking professional psychological assistance, such as therapy or counseling, can offer a secure setting where people can communicate their emotions and get advice on managing the psychological components of the illness.

Assistance Networks

Creating a solid support system is essential for those with genital herpes. Support networks, family, and friends can provide encouragement, understanding, and empathy. Developing relationships with people who have gone through comparable things helps people feel less alone and more like a part of the community. Support groups can offer persons with genital herpes a forum to talk about their struggles and victories as well as helpful guidance and emotional support.

Relationships And Disclosure

When a person has genital herpes, managing relationships requires addressing intimacy and transparency. Healthy relationships depend on open communication, and people need to think carefully about whether and how to tell partners they are herpes positive. This section examines the intricacies of disclosure and talks about how dating and intimacy are affected by it.

Speaking With Partners

Giving a spouse a diagnosis of genital herpes necessitates thoughtful thought and dialogue. It's crucial to have frank discussions about herpes, how it spreads, and ways to lower your risk. Gaining a partner's understanding and acceptance can be facilitated by building trust and giving truthful facts. Involving partners in decisions about their sexual health, addressing concerns, and providing information all contribute to a collaborative approach to managing sexual health within the framework of relationships.

Intimacy And Dating

Having genital herpes might cause anxiety when it comes to intimacy and relationships. People may struggle with deciding whether and how to tell a new partner that they are herpes positive.

The dating process can be made more difficult by the dread of rejection and shame. It's critical to approach dating with integrity and honesty, placing a strong emphasis on consent and open communication. Those with genital herpes can build happy, healthy personal relationships by practicing safe sex, educating oneself and others about the infection, and being aware of potential triggers.

there are psychological and physical difficulties associated with having genital herpes. Support groups and coping mechanisms are essential for assisting people in handling the emotional components of the illness. Furthermore, managing relationships calls for honest disclosure, open communication, and the development of mutual understanding when it comes to dating and intimacy. People with genital herpes can manage the complications of this prevalent STI and strive toward leading fulfilled lives by treating the emotional and psychological aspects of the condition.

Faqs Regarding Genital Herpes

The herpes simplex virus (HSV) is the source of genital herpes, a sexually transmitted infection (STI). It causes severe physical agony as well as psychological misery when it appears as excruciating sores or blisters in the vaginal and anal regions.

When answering frequently asked questions about genital herpes, it is important to discuss the infection's characteristics, how it affects pregnancy, and why it is considered an STD.

Can You Cure Genital Herpes?

Is genital herpes curable? is one of the most commonly asked questions regarding it. Regretfully, genital herpes has no known cure as of this writing in medical literature. It is well known that the herpes simplex virus can cause latent infections in nerve cells, which makes it difficult to completely eradicate from the body.

Antiviral drugs including valacyclovir, famciclovir, and acyclovir are frequently administered to treat symptoms, lessen the likelihood of transmission, and lessen the frequency of outbreaks.

These drugs don't completely eradicate the virus, but they can be useful in managing it.

Although there are ongoing studies looking into novel therapeutic approaches and possible vaccines, a permanent solution is still unattainable.

What Impact Does Genital Herpes Have On Conception?

Because genital herpes can affect both the developing fetus and the expectant woman, its effects on pregnancy are a serious matter.

To monitor and minimize any hazards, pregnant individuals with genital herpes should get specialized prenatal care. The main worry is that the baby could contract neonatal herpes, a virus that is spread to newborns during childbirth.

If there are active lesions at the time of delivery, there is a greater chance of transmission. It could be advised to deliver the baby via cesarean section to lower this risk. Antiviral drugs may also be recommended during pregnancy in order to reduce viral activity and lower the likelihood of a breakout close to the time of delivery.

Healthcare professionals must collaborate closely with pregnant patients who have genital herpes in order to create a complete plan that protects the health of the mother and the unborn child.

Do Sexually Transmitted Diseases (Stds) Include Herpes?

Without a doubt, herpes is considered a sexually transmitted infection (STD). Genital herpes is frequently caused by the herpes simplex virus, more precisely HSV-2, which is mainly spread through intercourse. Nonetheless, oral-genital contact can also transfer HSV-1, which is usually linked to oral herpes, to the genital region. Direct skin-to-skin contact with an infected individual can transfer the virus, especially during vaginal, anal, or oral intercourse. Although they can lessen the chance of transmission, barrier techniques like condoms and dental dams do not provide 100% protection. The frequency of genital herpes emphasizes how crucial safe sexual behaviors and honest communication between partners are. Preventing the spread of genital herpes and reducing its impact on sexual health need education regarding the biology of the virus, its mechanisms of transmission, and the importance of routine testing.

answering often asked concerns regarding genital herpes entails examining its categorization as an STD, its inability to cure, and its impact on pregnancy. The fact that there is now no cure emphasizes how crucial it is to keep researching possible treatments and safeguards. To reduce the chances of neonatal herpes, pregnant women must receive thorough prenatal care and work in tandem with healthcare specialists. Last but not least, the fact that herpes is now classified as an STD highlights the need of safe sexual behaviors as well as the necessity for public awareness and education to stop its spread.

CHAPTER EIGHT
FALLACIES AND MISUNDERSTANDINGS

Many myths and misconceptions about genital herpes, which is brought on by the herpes simplex virus (HSV), lead to stigma and misunderstanding. Dispelling these myths is essential to disseminating correct information and lessening the condition's negative social effects.

Oral Sex And Herpes

A common misconception regarding genital herpes is the idea that genital-to-genital contact is the only way the virus may spread. In actuality, oral-genital contact can spread the HSV virus and cause genital herpes. This misunderstanding frequently results from the distinction between types 1 and 2 of the herpes simplex virus (HSV-1). HSV-1 can transmit from the mouth to the genitalia, which is why it is commonly linked to oral herpes.

The same is true for HSV-2, which is sometimes associated with genital herpes but can also cause oral infections when it comes into contact with the genitalia.

Preventive measures require an understanding of the potential for oral intercourse to transmit genital herpes. The risk of transmission can be greatly decreased by using condoms or dental dams during sexual activity. Dispelling the notion that oral sex is not a route of transmission for genital herpes requires education about the dual capacity of both HSV strains to infect both oral and genital regions.

Restroom Seats And Herpes

There's also a common misconception about getting herpes from using toilet seats. This false belief is the result of ignorance regarding the virus's route of spread. The main way that herpes is spread is by direct skin-to-skin contact with an affected area when the virus is shedding.

The virus cannot thrive on inanimate surfaces like toilet seats because it is brittle outside the body.

It's imperative to debunk the misconception that herpes can spread via toilet seats in order to reduce needless stress and anxiety. Informed public health education can benefit from highlighting the necessity of direct skin contact during viral shedding and the virus's incapacity to proliferate on surfaces.

With this understanding, people can stop worrying unnecessarily about getting herpes from common surfaces and instead concentrate on doing preventive actions like washing their hands frequently.

Herpes And Informal Interaction

The idea that genital herpes can be easily spread through casual, non-intimate contact is a common misperception about the condition. Actually, for HSV to spread, the virus needs to come into direct contact with mucous membranes or skin breaches. There is very little chance of herpes transmission during informal encounters including handshakes, hugs, and sharing of personal goods.

It's imperative to debunk this myth in order to lessen the stigma attached to genital herpes. Fighting the unwarranted fear and prejudice frequently aimed towards people with herpes is made easier by highlighting the significance of direct, personal touch for transmission. Educating people on the low danger of casual contact advances correct knowledge of the virus and fosters a more sympathetic and supportive social climate.

eradicating widespread misconceptions about genital herpes is essential to creating a culture that is more empathetic and knowledgeable.

Dispelling myths about oral sex, using toilet seats, and casual contact gives people the information they need to make wise choices, lessen stigma, and show support for persons who have genital herpes. Disseminating correct information should be given top priority in public health programs to counter false information and ultimately create a community that is more accepting and understanding.

CHAPTER NINE
PROSPECTIVE ROUTES

For us to further understand the virus and develop treatment alternatives, genital herpes research must continue. Scholars are rigorously investigating a range of topics, including the molecular mechanisms underlying the herpes simplex virus (HSV) and the creation of innovative therapeutic strategies. The goal of advances in diagnostic instruments is to improve accurate diagnosis and early detection. This includes looking into precise and sensitive molecular markers that can help diagnose herpes more accurately.

Furthermore, a concentrated effort is being made to understand the intricate relationship that exists between the virus and the host immune system. This entails researching possible immunomodulatory tactics, identifying important immunological pathways, and researching the immune response to HSV infection.

Developing successful treatment approaches requires an understanding of the immunological host-virus interaction.

In addition to its molecular and immunological components, research on the psychological effects of genital herpes is still in progress.

The goal of research is to create specialized solutions to support those who have genital herpes by examining the psychological and emotional effects of having the condition. Herpes research takes a holistic approach, including social, psychological, and medical aspects to solve the complex issues surrounding this virus.

Improvements In Medical Care

Progress in the management of genital herpes is the main focus of current investigations.

The cornerstone of treatment for a long time has been antiviral drugs, and scientists are always looking for novel antiviral agents and treatment plans to improve effectiveness and lessen adverse effects. To address the problem of drug resistance and enhance treatment outcomes, combination therapies—which combine several antiviral medications—are now being researched.

Developing targeted treatments with the goal of sabotaging particular viral life cycle stages is another line of inquiry.

This comprises drugs that block the entrance, replication, and assembly of viruses, providing a more focused and possibly less harmful course of therapy. In order to create treatments that alter host responses to prevent viral replication, research is also being done to uncover host variables that contribute to HSV infection.

Research on immunomodulatory therapies for genital herpes is an intriguing new area.

To restrict viral replication, strategies that strengthen the host immune response or alter immunological pathways are being researched. Research into therapeutic vaccines, which aim to elicit a strong and long-lasting immune response against HSV, is also very promising.

Advances In Vaccination

In the field, creating a vaccine against genital herpes is still a top focus. Numerous vaccination strategies, such as DNA vaccines, subunit vaccines, and live attenuated vaccines, are being actively investigated by researchers. Vaccines that have been live-attenuated are designed to minimize disease risk and elicit a protective immune response. Whereas DNA vaccines introduce viral DNA to trigger an immune response, subunit vaccinations concentrate on particular viral proteins to produce immunity.

Preclinical research and early-stage clinical trials have demonstrated the potential of a number of vaccine candidates.

The goals of these contenders are to offer medicinal and prophylactic advantages. Preventive vaccines try to shield people from infection from the outset, whereas therapeutic vaccines try to lessen the frequency and intensity of repeated outbreaks.

The ability to provide long-lasting immunity, managing viral diversity, and guaranteeing safety, particularly in populations with pre-existing diseases, are challenges in the creation of vaccines. Working together, academic institutions, pharmaceutical firms, and government agencies will be essential to overcome these obstacles and moving vaccine candidates forward through thorough clinical trials.

Awareness And Advocacy

Campaigns for advocacy and awareness are essential in dispelling the myths surrounding genital herpes, disseminating correct information, and providing support to those who are infected. In order to increase public knowledge of the prevalence, transmission, and consequences of genital herpes, advocacy activities involve interacting with legislators, medical experts, and the general public.

Campaigns for public health seek to debunk misconceptions about herpes and highlight the value of screening, education, and honest communication. In order to create a supportive environment where people feel comfortable seeking medical assistance and telling partners they are infected; it is imperative that efforts be made to lessen the stigma attached to genital herpes.

Furthermore, advocacy encompasses the promotion of comprehensive sex education that includes information about STDs and guarantees fair access to healthcare services. This entails de-stigmatizing conversations about sexual health and promoting frequent HSV-1 and HSV-2 testing.

A comprehensive strategy to genital herpes awareness and support requires collaboration between advocacy groups, healthcare practitioners, and legislators.

Advocacy programs assist in removing obstacles to genital herpes diagnosis, treatment, and general well-being by promoting a more knowledgeable and caring society.

CONCLUSION

genital herpes is a common and clinically serious STD that has a wide range of effects on both the health of those who have it and the general public. Healthcare practitioners, researchers, and policymakers must have a thorough understanding of the epidemiology, pathophysiology, clinical symptoms, diagnosis, treatment, and preventive initiatives. Research, diagnostics, and treatment developments are still influencing how we treat genital herpes, providing promise for better results, lower transmission rates, and higher quality of life for those living with this difficult illness.

The ongoing endeavor to decipher the intricacies of genital herpes underscores the importance of a comprehensive and interdisciplinary strategy in tackling this worldwide health issue.